SEXY FITNESS ARMS

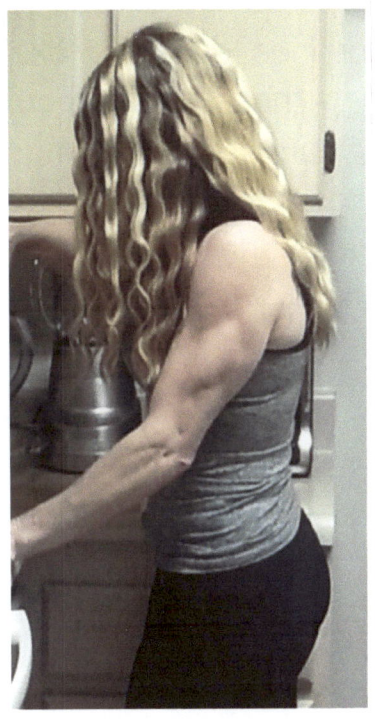

I0417652

Copyright © 2017

By Kathleen (Lil Kat) Jones

Sexy Fitness Arms
By Kathleen (Lil Kat) Jones

.

Sexy Fitness Arms is intended to be used for general guidelines only. No exercise of any kind, including those in this book, should be attempted without first consulting with a doctor first. The outcome results are not foreseen or guaranteed and individual results can and will vary depending on many factors not addressed in this book.

Sexy Fitness Arms
By Kathleen (Lil Kat) Jones

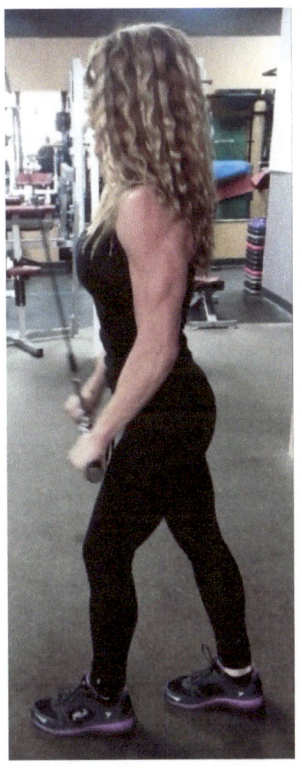

Sexy Fitness Arms is intended to be used for general guidelines only and no exercise of any kind, including those in this book, should be attempted without first consulting with a doctor and determining your physical suitability for strenuous exercise. The results in the book are not guaranteed and individual results will vary depending on many factors not addressed in this book.

The Workout

Now let's train and start developing those sexy and fit arms.

Skull crushers
Standing barbell curls
Cable press downs (straight bar)
Dumbbell hammer curls
Body weight dips
Side laterals

TRICEPS (EXERCISE #1)
Skull Crushers

Now let's start training and let's begin with the all to famous skull crushers also known as kick-outs and let's load it with a fairly controllable weight using a straight bar. Make sure that you don't load this up with a over challenging weight as we will be doing 4 set of 25 repetitions for our triceps (the upper back part of the arm) with very little rest in between each set.

Sexy Fitness Arms
By Kathleen (Lil Kat) Jones

The goal is to perform the first set of 25 repetitions and take a short rest of 60 seconds. Then immediately begin the second set of 25 repetitions and repeat the 60 seconds of rest. Then begin set number three and repeat until you have successfully completed all four sets of 25 repetitions, equaling a total of 100 repetitions.

Now the reality is that most of you will need to stop and rest in the middle of the set. This is normal until you get your body conditioned to a higher level and then you'll be able to conduct all four sets with stopping any longer than the 60 seconds specified in between each set. For those who do need to rest in the middle of the 25 repetition set, try not to rest for longer than 15-30 seconds and resume where you left off at in your count, until you reach 25 repetitions.

Sexy Fitness Arms
By Kathleen (Lil Kat) Jones

TRICEPS (EXERCISE #1)
Skull Crushers 4 set's of 25 repetitions
100 repetitions total.

Grip the bar with thumbs on top.

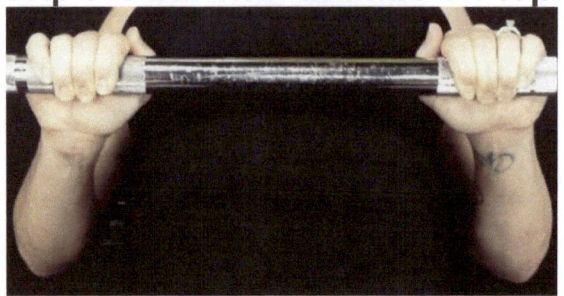

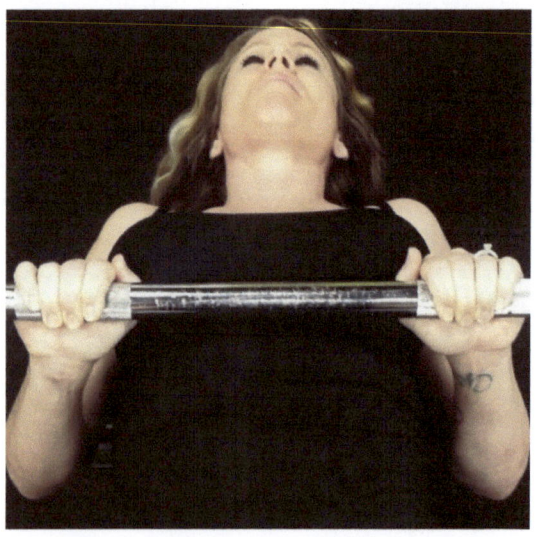

Rest on chest if or when needed.

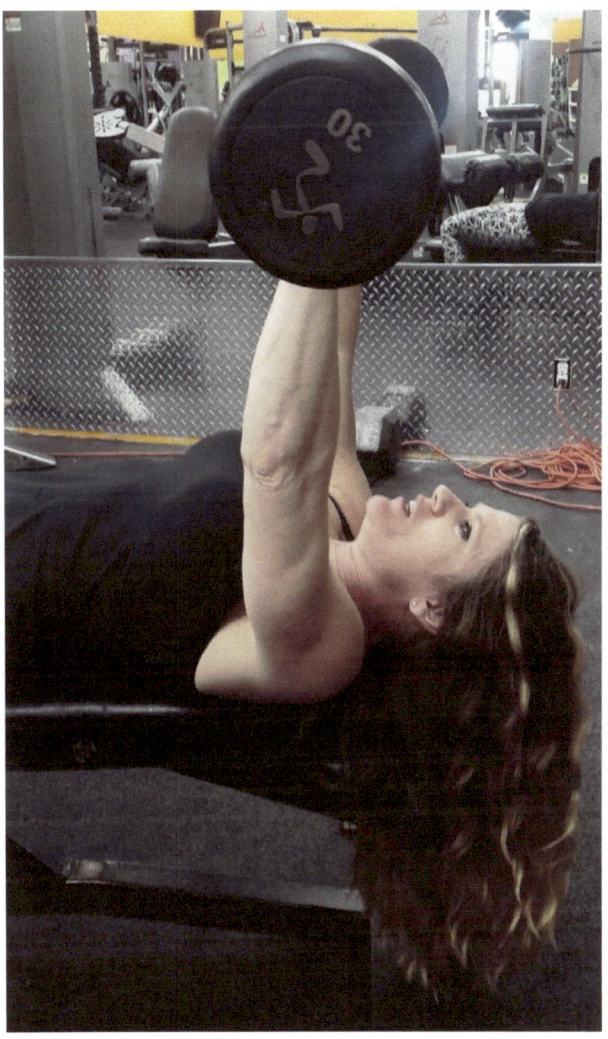

At the top of this movement, begin to inhale just before bringing the weight downward.

Sexy Fitness Arms
By Kathleen (Lil Kat) Jones

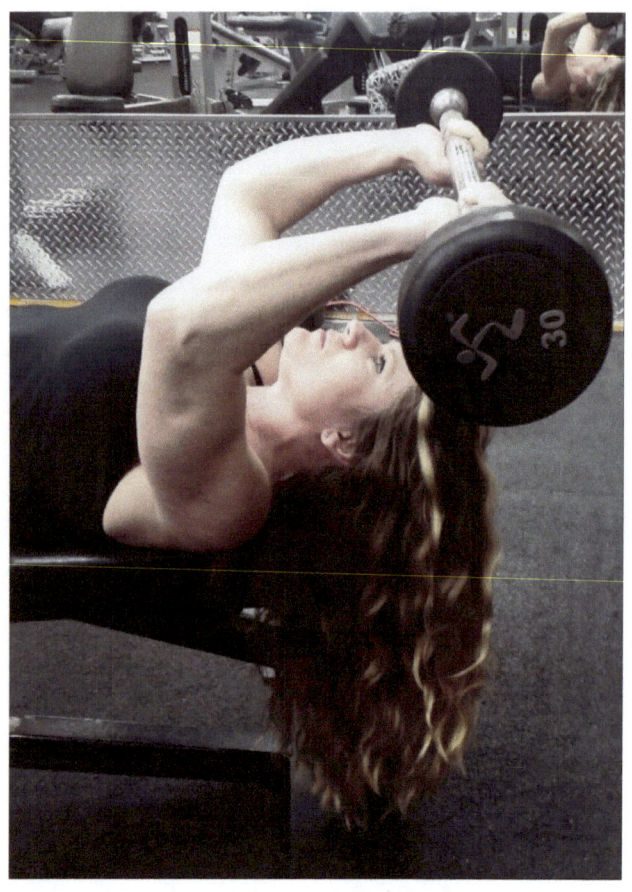

Continue inhaling as you're bringing the weight downward. Also keep a tight hand grip on the bar, as this will give you more power as you're performing this movement.

Sexy Fitness Arms
By Kathleen (Lil Kat) Jones

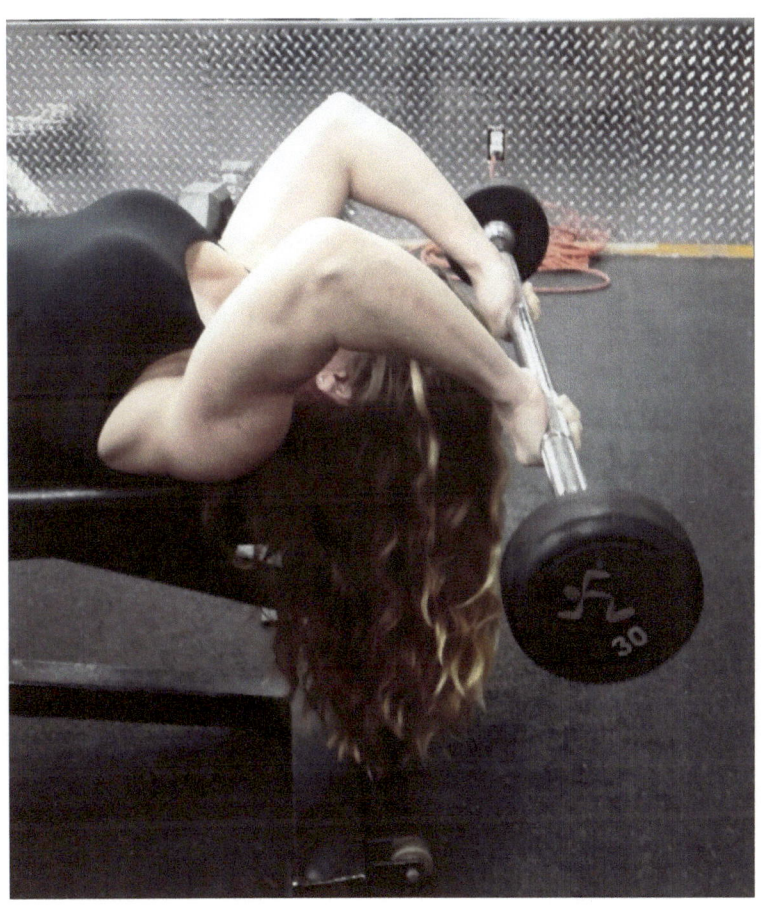

Now just before powering the weight upward begin to exhale, but don't fully exhale until you are at the top/completion of the repetition.

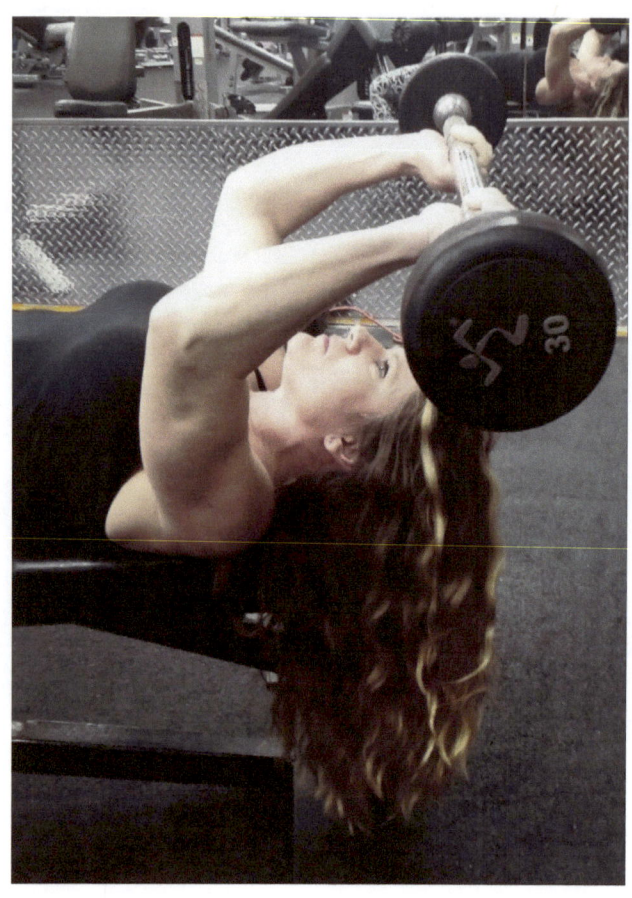

Continue to blow out (exhaling) as you are bringing the weight back upward.

Sexy Fitness Arms
By Kathleen (Lil Kat) Jones

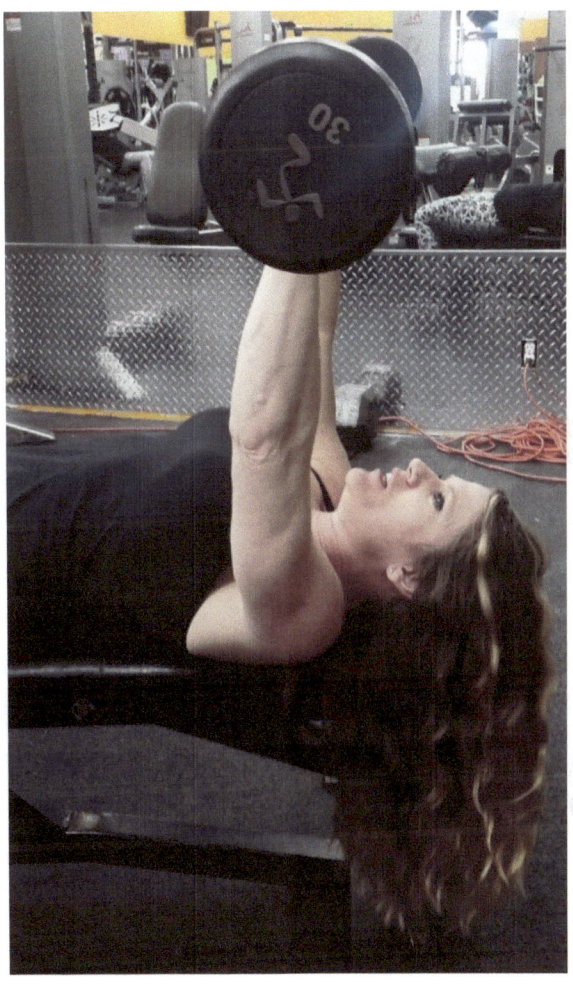

As you return to the top of this movement fully exhale and repeat for 25 reps for 4 sets, 100 reps in total.

Remember to only rest for 60 seconds in between each set.

Sexy Fitness Arms
By Kathleen (Lil Kat) Jones

Standing Barbell Curls

Now that our triceps are full of blood with a good pump, let's now focus on our biceps with a traditional straight bar standing barbell curl, using a standard shoulder width grip. Select a weight that you know is light weight enough for you complete 25 repetitions straight for 4 sets, making your total count, 100 repetitions, just as we did above with the skull crushers.

Remember try your best not to rest for longer than 60 seconds between sets. This will be tough but you can do it. If you start to tire do as many as you can and split the reps if needed into repetitions of 5 for example if you are rep 10 and you decide you need to rest, don't set the weight down "but" take a breather and then make a 5 rep commitment and go for 15 reps and so on, until you complete the entire 25 repetitions. Ok we're not done with our training yet so let's get back to training.

Sexy Fitness Arms
By Kathleen (Lil Kat) Jones

Standard hand grip.

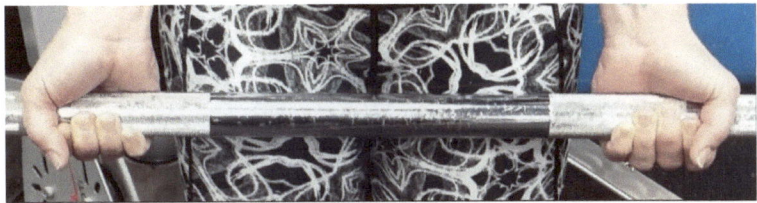

Here we'll use a traditional standard hand grip as we perform the standing barbell curl. By gripping the bar tightly you may find that you will discover additional strength to perform this exercise. We also will want to focus on correct breathing patterns, which will be explained in the photos below each illustrated photo. Breathing properly will definitely maximize your ability to complete each set of 25 repetitions, just as improper breathing will definitely hinder your full potential in performing this exercise.

Sexy Fitness Arms
By Kathleen (Lil Kat) Jones

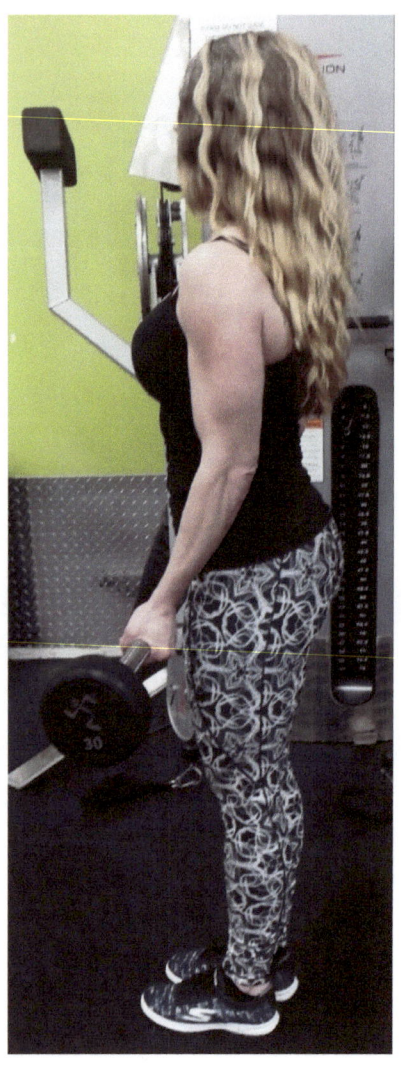

Take a deep breath, filling up your lungs
and just before curling upward begin to
exhale.

Sexy Fitness Arms
By Kathleen (Lil Kat) Jones

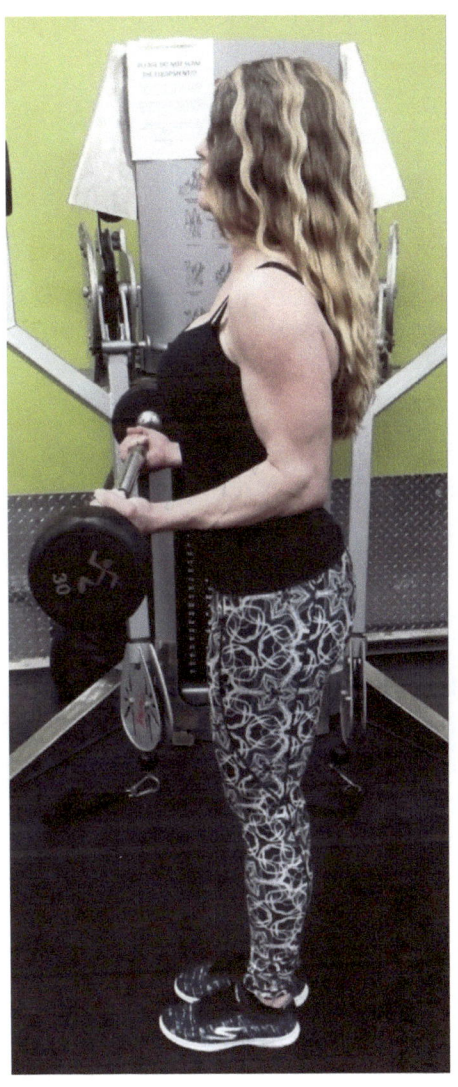

Continue to blow out (exhaling) as you are
curling the weight upward.

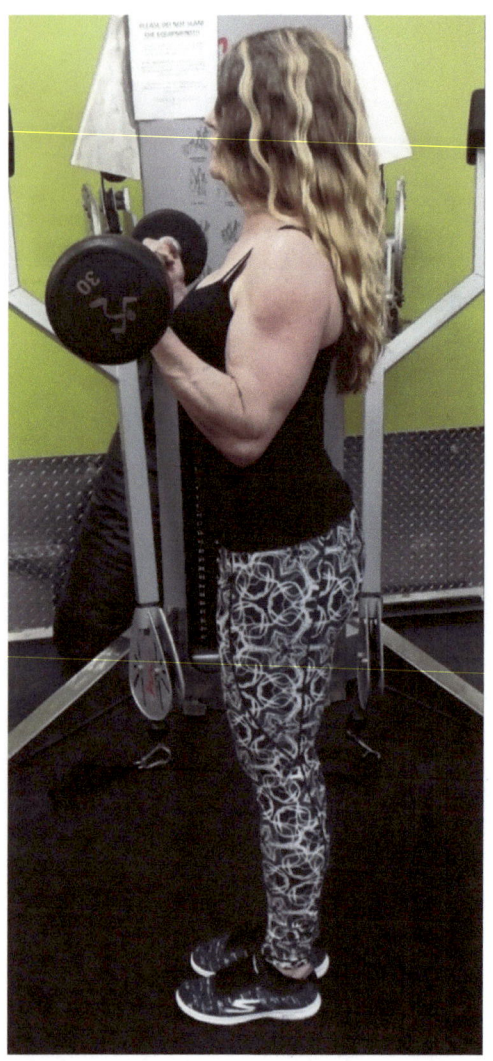

Now fully exhale at the top and repeat for 25 reps. Do 4 sets of 25reps for a total of 100 repetitions.

Cable Press Downs

Now let's return back to our triceps and let's now do another 4 sets of 25 repetitions with the exact same rest periods as above 60 second in between if training alone and if training with a workout partner rest only while your training partner is performing their set of 25 reps. By now I'm sure at this point you can see the importance of your mind being set for achievement as this is going to a game of mental strength as well as physical strength.

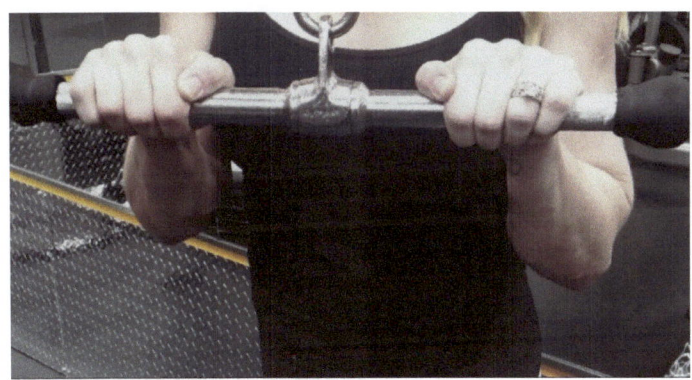

Thumbs on top.

17

Sexy Fitness Arms
By Kathleen (Lil Kat) Jones

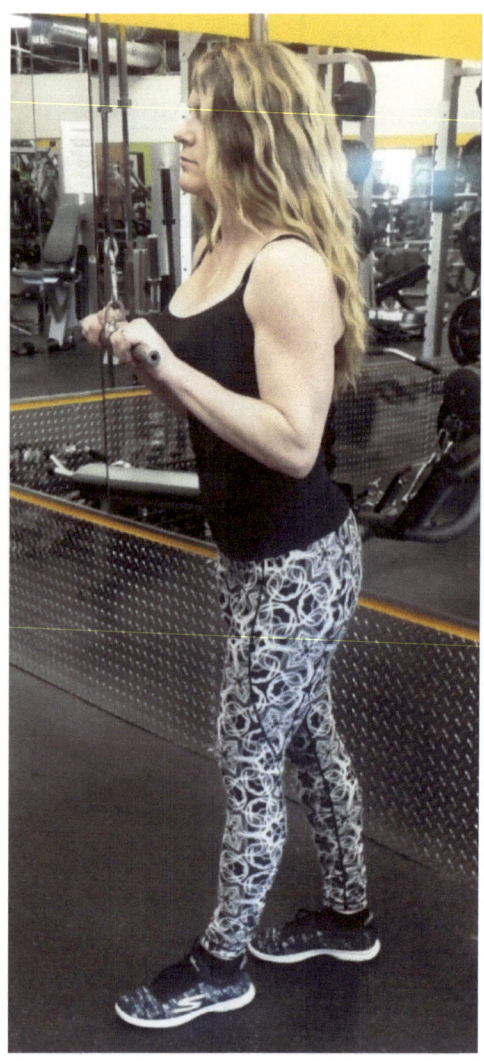

Lean slightly inward towards the cable, take a deep breath (side view) and just before pressing downward, begin to exhale.

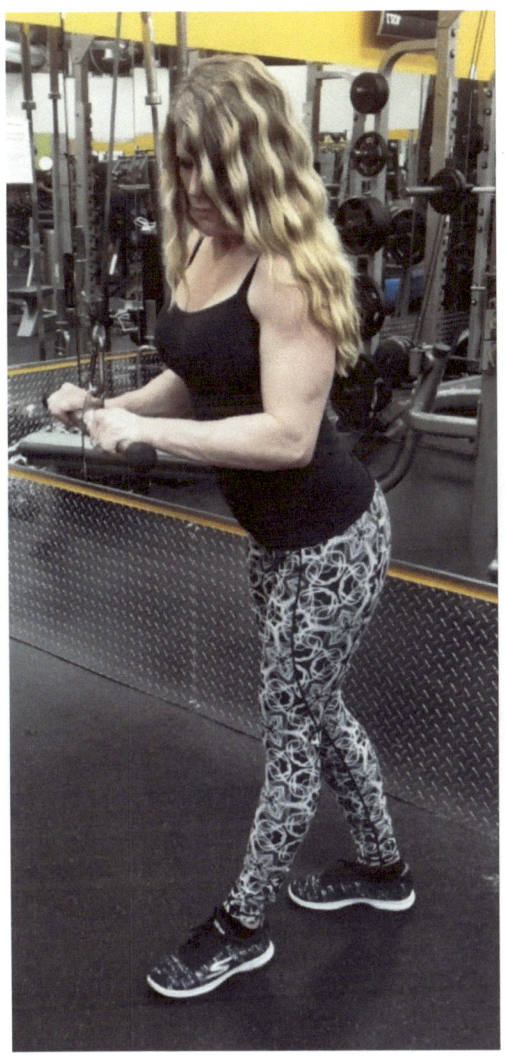

Continue exhaling (blowing out) as you're pressing the cable straight bar downward.

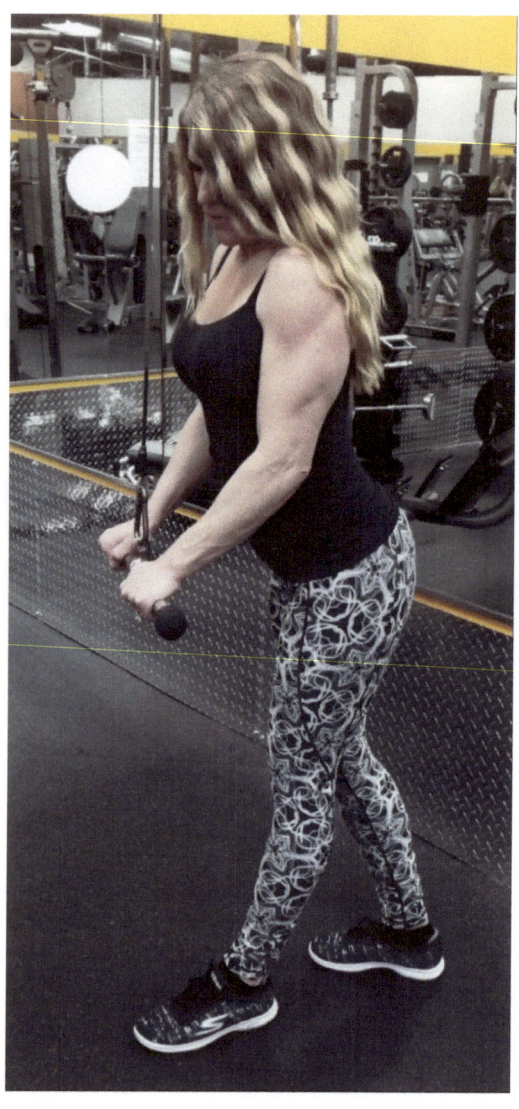

¾ of the way down still exhaling (blowing out) as you're pressing downward.

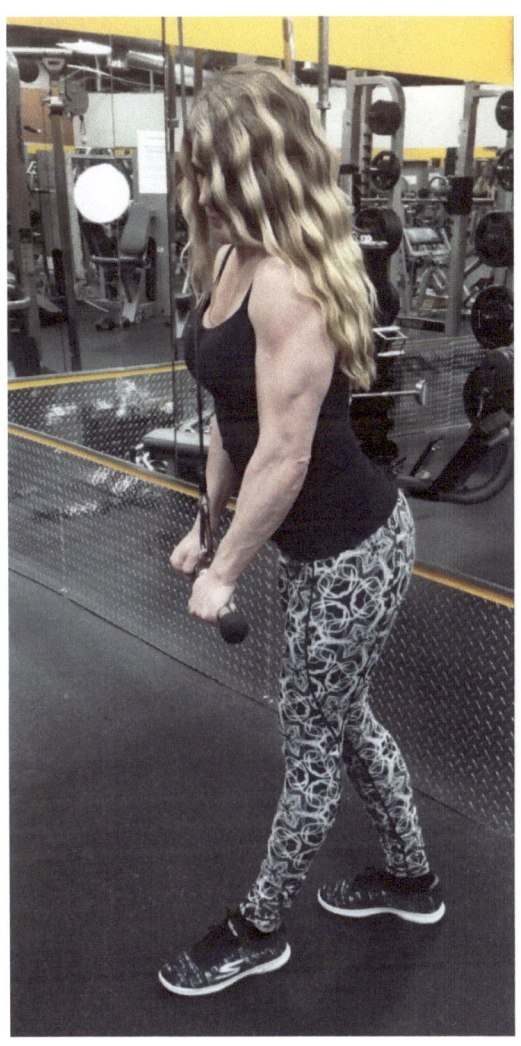

Fully exhale at the bottom and begin inhaling as you're returning to the original start position and repeat.

Dumbbell Hammer Curls

Now let's return for one more set of biceps and let's do a set of dumbbell hammer curls standing or sitting the choice is yours, and let's do another 4 sets of 25 reps for a total of 100 repetitions. Again only take a 60 second rest between sets unless you are training with a workout partner. Then only rest while they perform their set of 25 reps. Make each set of 25 repetitions a challenge.

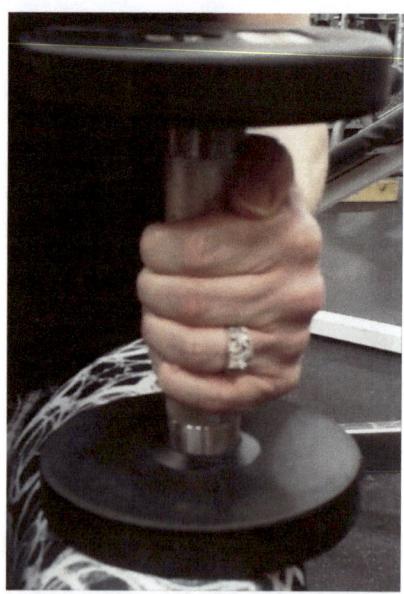

Hammer Curls Hand Position

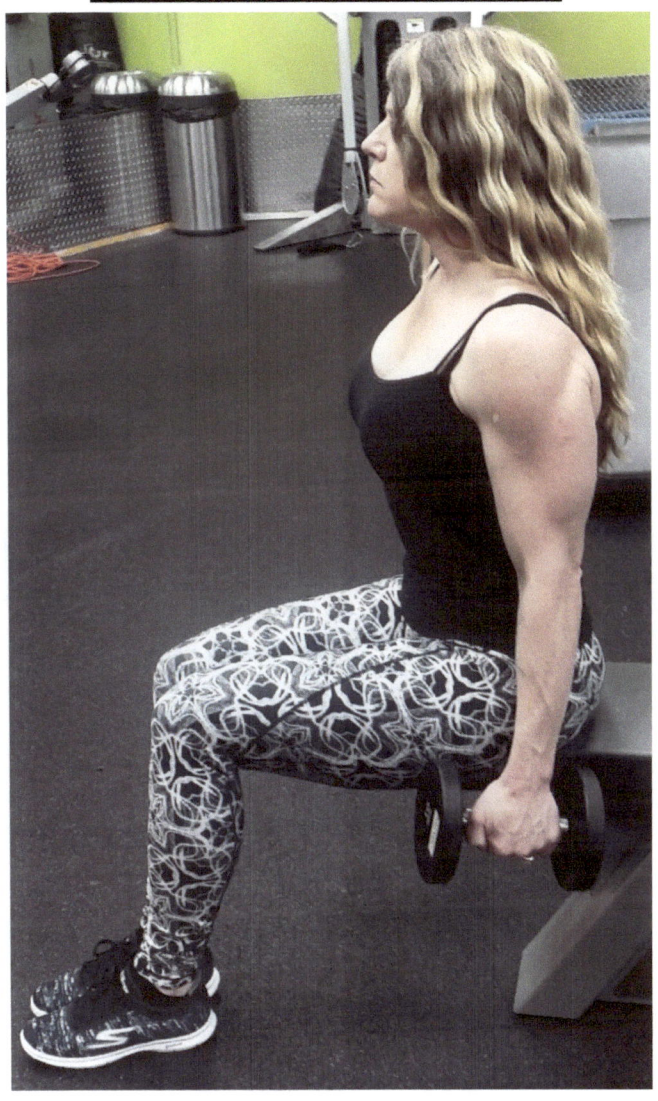

Take a deep breath and just before curling upward begin to slowly blow out.

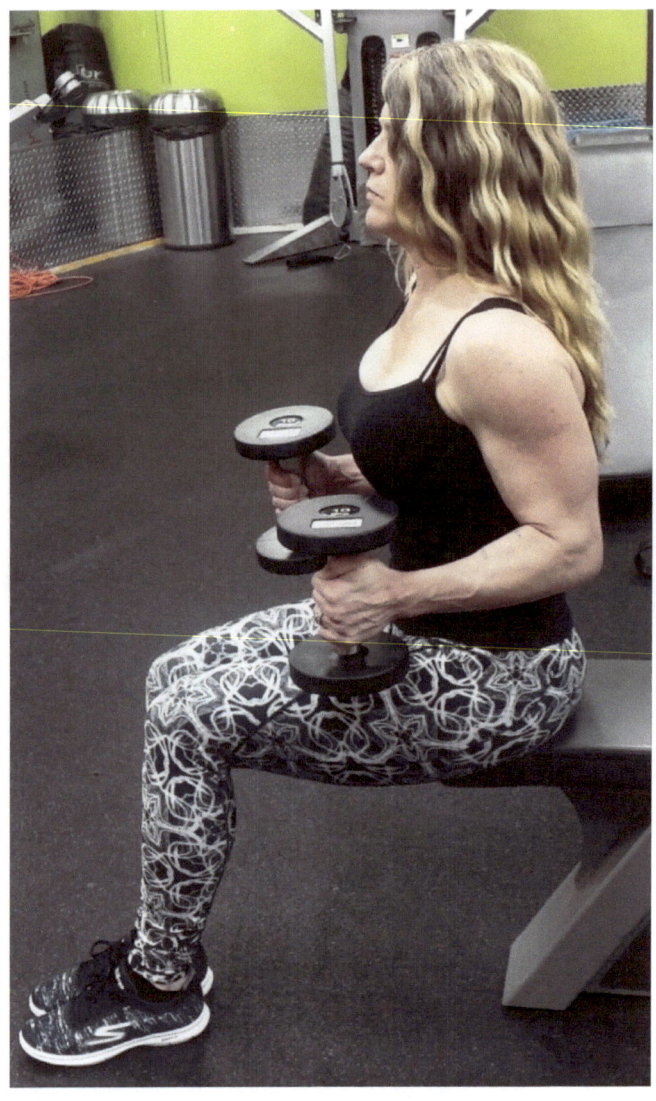

Continue blowing outward as you're curling the weight upward.

Sexy Fitness Arms
By Kathleen (Lil Kat) Jones

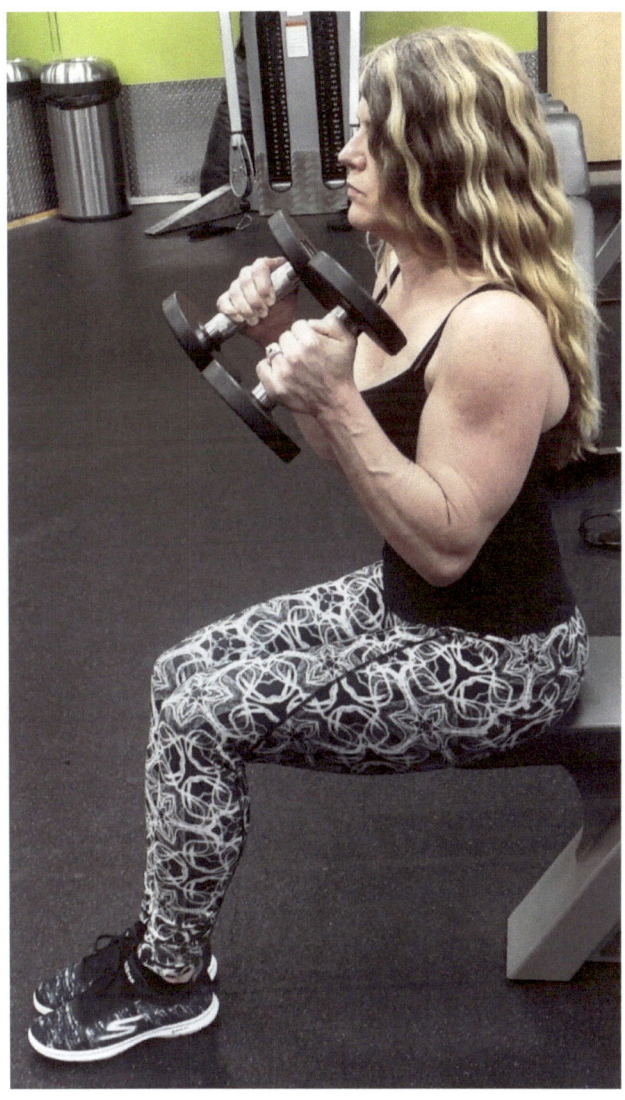

Fully exhale at the top of the movement and repeat. Do 4 sets of 25 reps for a total of 100 reps.

Body Weight Dips

Now for the final exercise of the day, we will move to body weight dips, here we will also do another 4 sets of 25 reps for a total of 100 repetitions. Make sure that at the bottom of each repetition we are going deep enough to really stress the triceps (backside of the upper arm) for change.

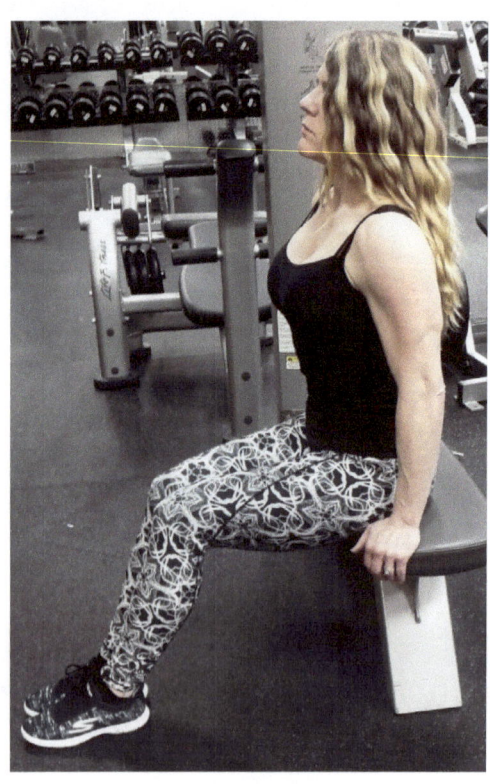

<u>Sexy Fitness Arms</u>
<u>By Kathleen (Lil Kat) Jones</u>

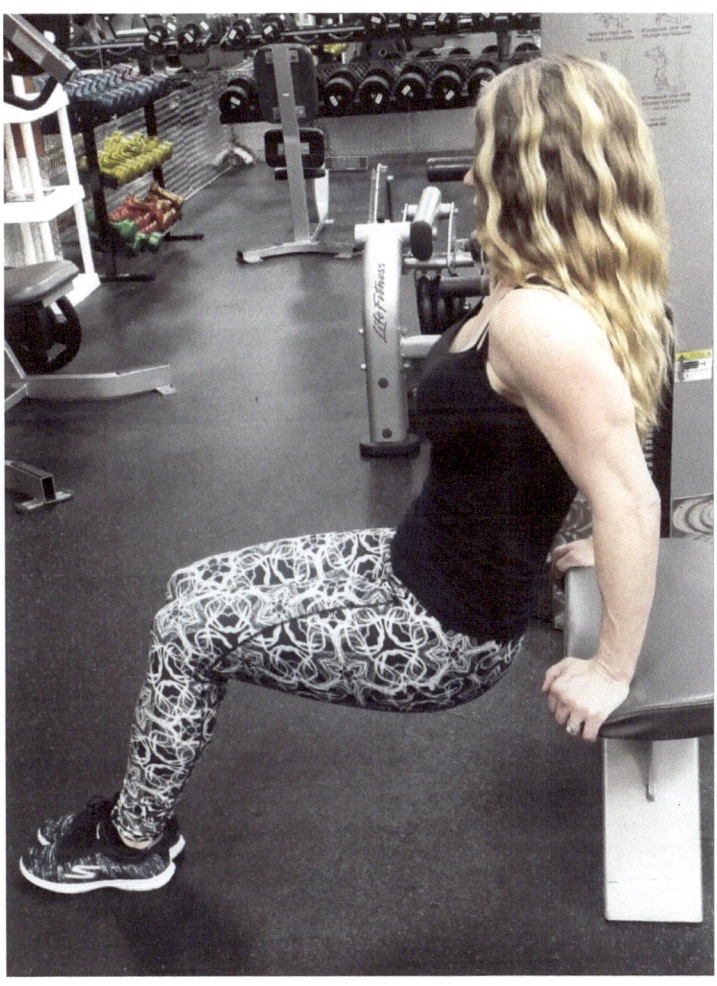

At the start position (shown above) begin to inhale as you are lowering yourself downward.

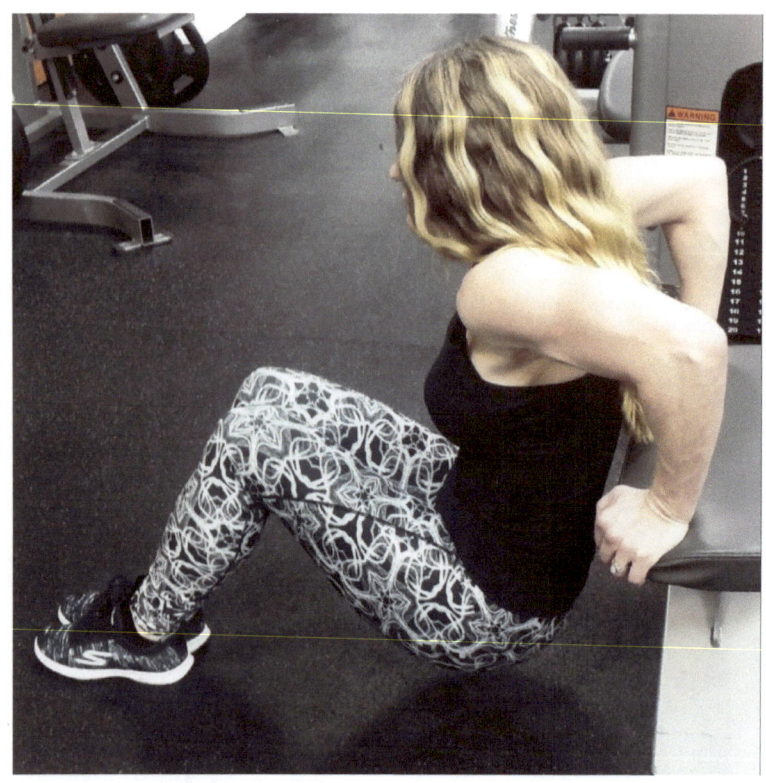

Continue to inhale as you are lowering your body downward.

Sexy Fitness Arms
By Kathleen (Lil Kat) Jones

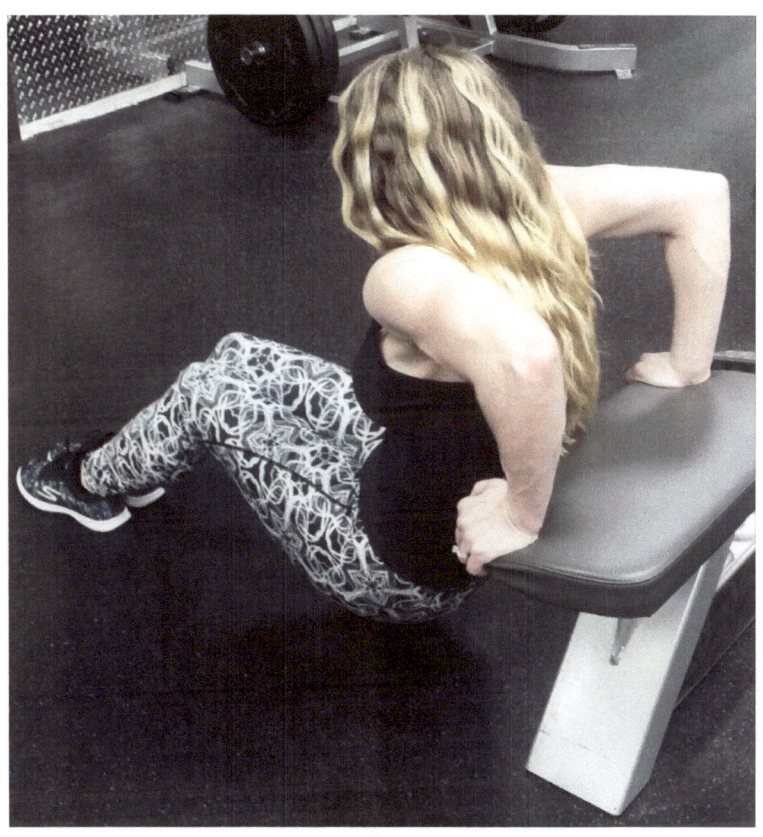

Now begin to blow out (exhale) as you are now beginning to press your body upward. Notice how the shoulder has dropped slightly below the elbow.

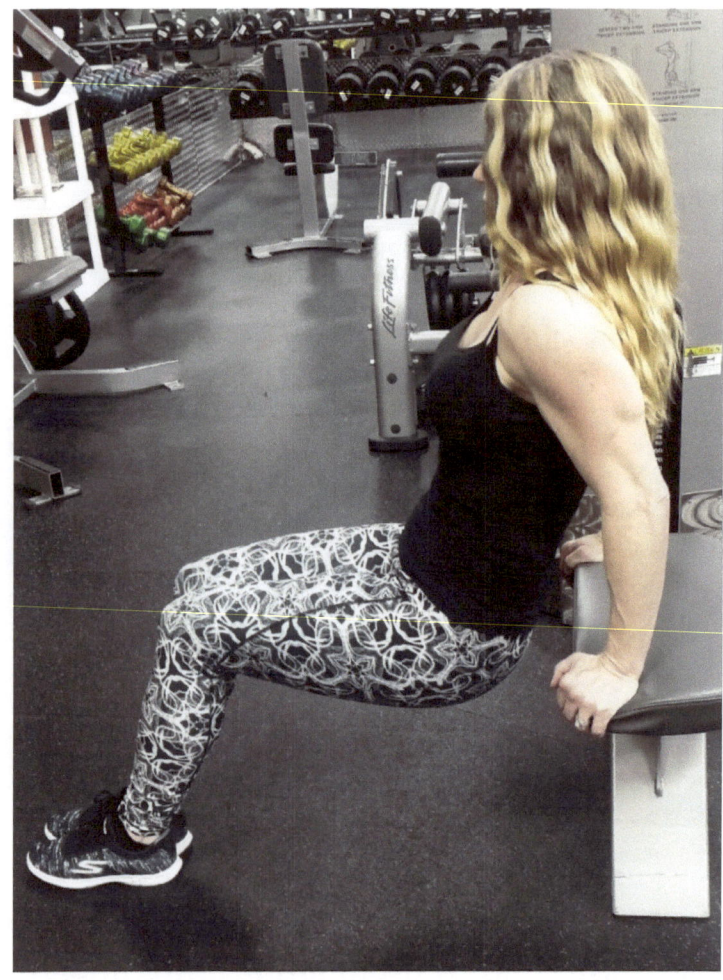

Fully exhale at the "top" of the movement and begin inhaling just before beginning the downward movement again.

Sexy Fitness Arms
By Kathleen (Lil Kat) Jones

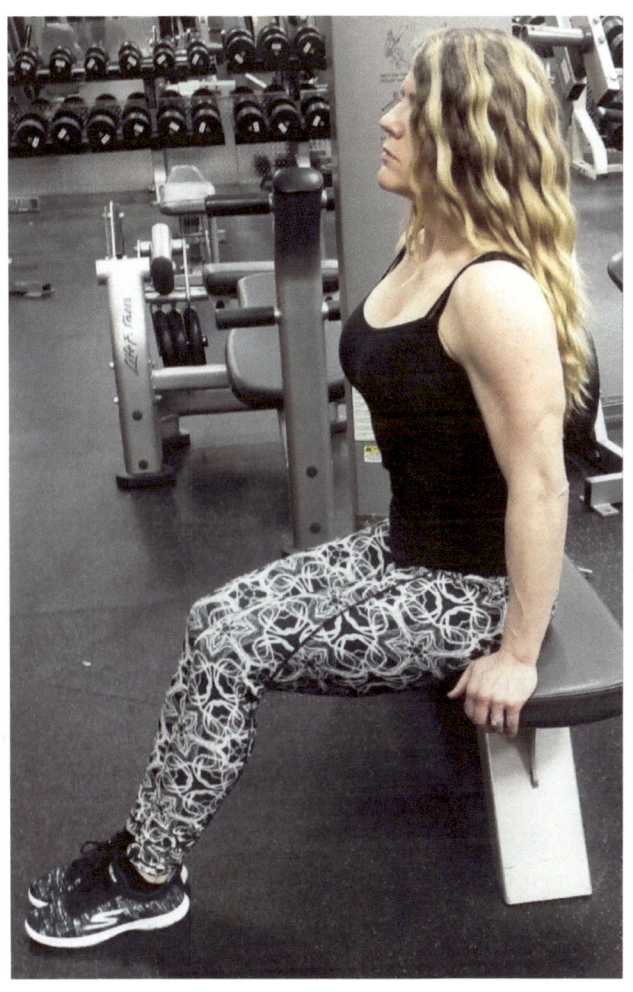

Do 4 sets of 25 repetitions for a total of 100 repetitions. Make sure to rest for "only" 60 seconds in between each set.

Sexy Fitness Arms
By Kathleen (Lil Kat) Jones

Side Laterals

We will now do side laterals as the final exercise towards developing sexy fit arms. Side laterals are a shoulder (Side Deltoid) exercise that will change the look of any arm when performed correctly on a regular basis. This is an exercise that will separate the shoulders and arms with a nice athletic detailed cut. This exercise alone will help get rid of what I call a "SHARM" you may be asking yourself what the heck is a "SHARM" it's when a person has a shoulder and arm smoothly blended together into one long looking muscle. This lack of definition alone will destroy the potential look of an awesome set of arms. This separation looks great on a woman and will simply enhance the overall appearance of a nice set of "sexy" arms. So as all the above exercises we will be doing 4 sets of 25 repetitions for a total of 100 repetitions. Make sure to do your best and only rest for no longer than 60 seconds in between each set. Ladies you "can" do this. NOTE: You can do this without any weights until you get stronger for additional resistance.

Sexy Fitness Arms
By Kathleen (Lil Kat) Jones

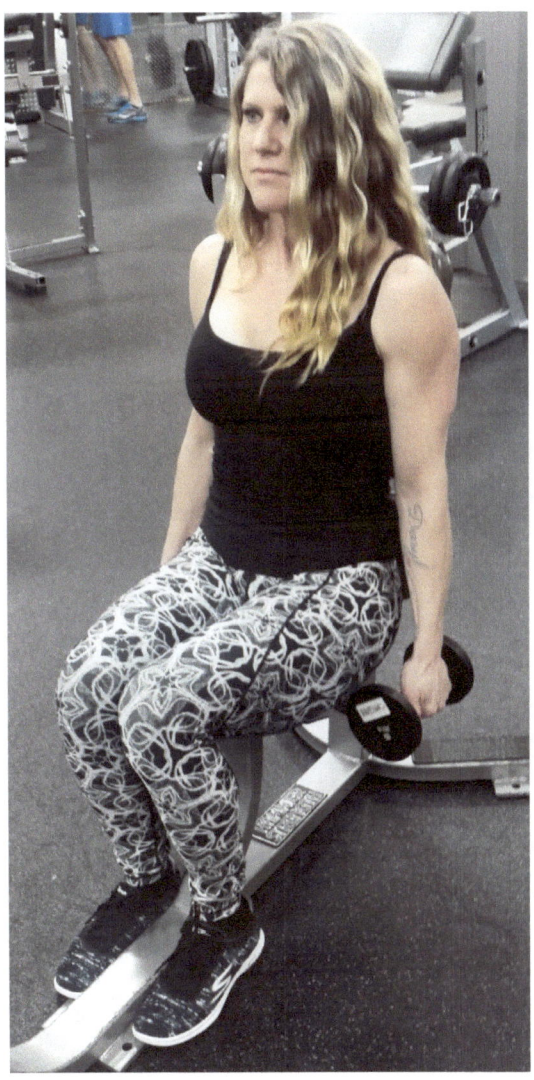

Starting position, take a deep breath before beginning the upward movement.

Sexy Fitness Arms
By Kathleen (Lil Kat) Jones

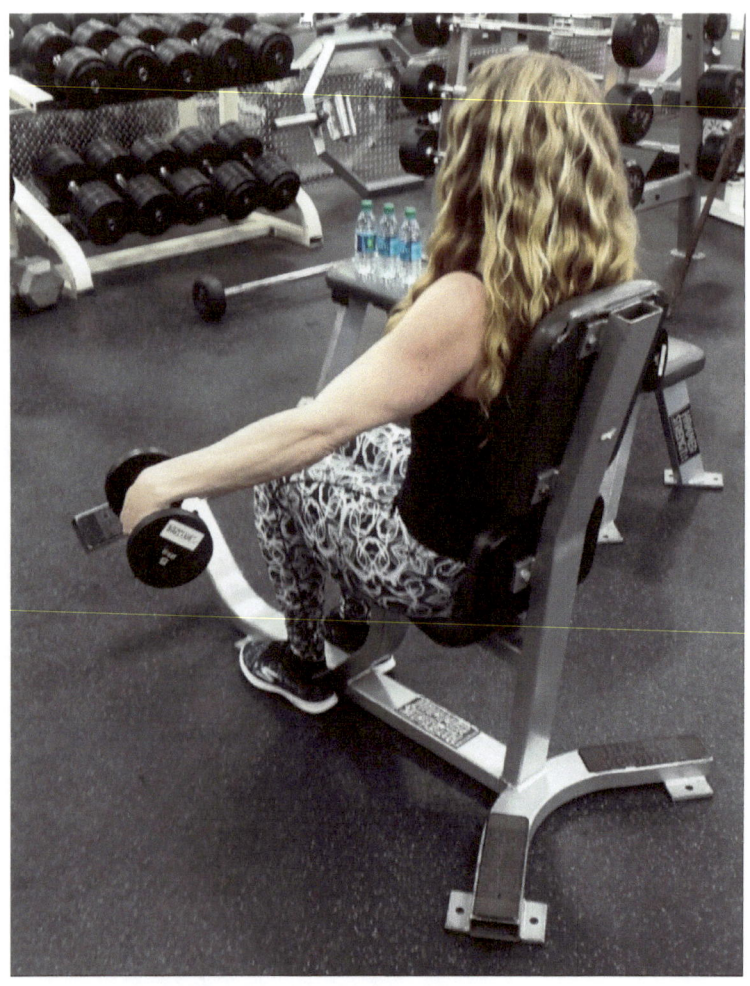

Exhale as you begin to lift upward. Lift up with a "wide" outward left to right reach, keeping the arms straight but without locking the joints.

Keep a slight bend in the elbow.

Sexy Fitness Arms
By Kathleen (Lil Kat) Jones

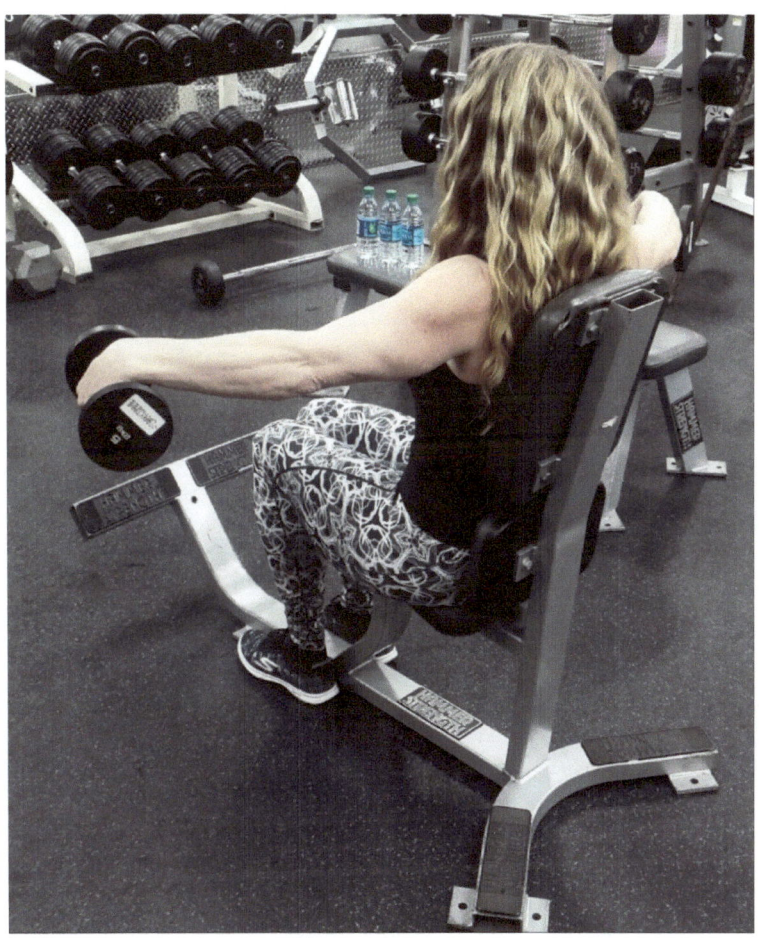

Continue to exhale as you are bringing the weights upward. Notice how the hands and wrist are bent downward, gripping the dumbbells in a hooking fashion.

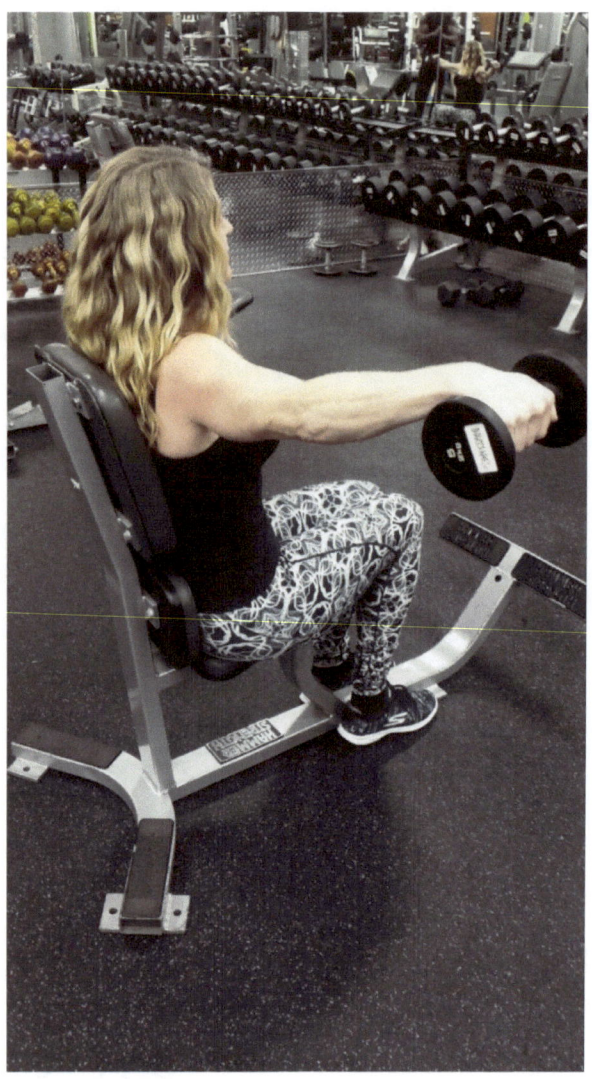

Here as we are now at the top of the movement, you'll notice how the elbow has come up equally as high as the shoulder.

Sexy Fitness Arms
By Kathleen (Lil Kat) Jones

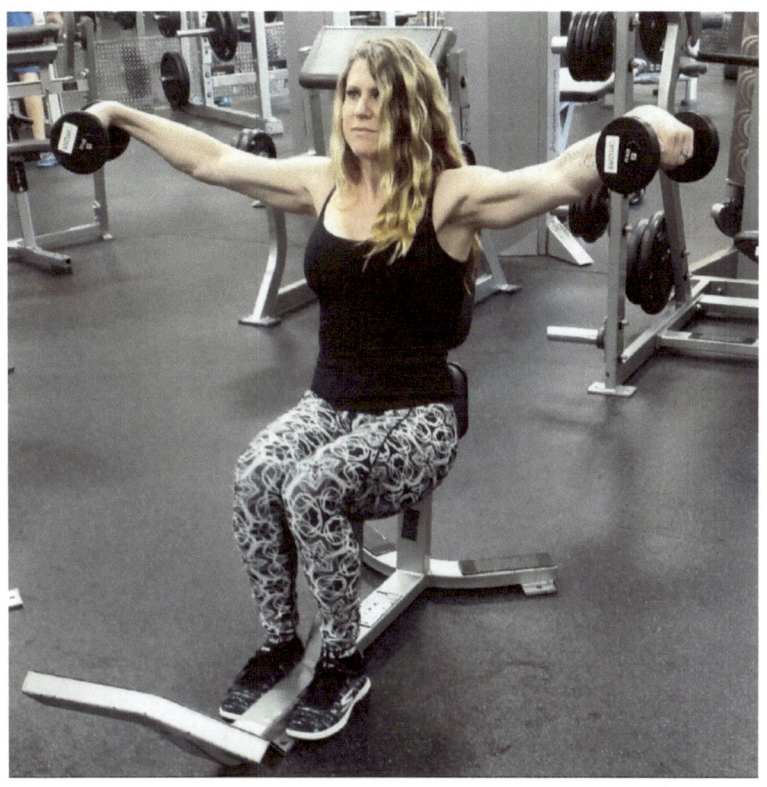

Fully exhale at the top of this movement and as you are now about to lower the arms in a controlled fashion, begin to inhale as the weight is being lowered. Again notice the bend in the wrist and the level of the elbow raising upward as high the shoulders themselves.

Sexy Fitness Arms
By Kathleen (Lil Kat) Jones

OBSTICLES

Success isn't measured by how many times you get knocked down, but rather how many times you get back up. Expect things to not go perfectly and don't get depressed or lose motivation simply because something unexpected happens. Always focus on the positive and don't brood on the negatives. You can overcome obstacles with some of these ideas:

If you miss a training day, simply start where you left off the very next day.

If you miss a scheduled meal don't eat two meals on the next scheduled eating time simply eat the next meal and go on from there.

If your time is limited beyond your normal control, don't miss the entire.

Sexy Fitness Arms
By Kathleen (Lil Kat) Jones

Workout, simply go into the gym and train with the available time you have (don't miss the entire training if possible).

These simple approaches that should aide you in successfully achieving your fitness goals, just know none of us are perfect but try to always give 110% effort toward your goals and I'm absolutely sure you'll be happy with your final results.

Train Hard and Then Train Harder!